EASY VEGAN RECIPES FOR DIABETES AND KIDNEY DISEASE

Plant-Based Recipes for Managing Diabetes and Kidney Disease (Includes 30 Day meal plans)

Dr Lily Morgan

COPYRIGHT PAGE

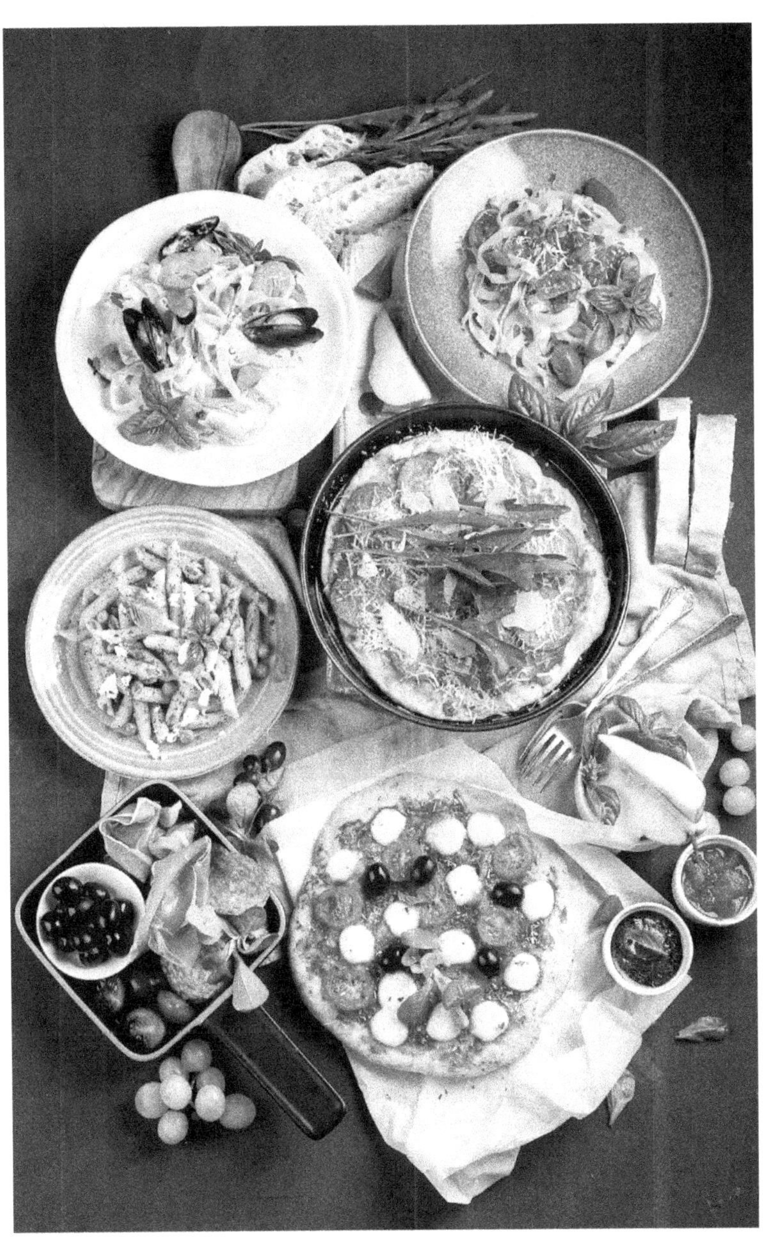

TABLE OF CONTENTS

Chapter 3: Lunch Recipes 38

Chapter 4: Dinner Recipes 55

Chapter 5: Snacks and Appetizers 74

INTRODUCTION

As we embark on a journey of exploration into the realm of culinary choices that cater to both diabetes and kidney health, while embracing the principles of a vegan lifestyle. The importance of such a dietary approach cannot be overstated, as it holds the potential to positively impact the well-being and quality of life for those facing these health challenges.

While many might initially view the idea of veganism as limited or restrictive, it is quite the contrary. The vast array of plant-based ingredients, herbs, and spices available opens a world of possibilities for creating delicious and satisfying dishes that cater to diverse palates. Whether you are a seasoned vegan, a curious newcomer, or someone seeking dietary changes for health reasons, this guide promises to deliver exciting recipes that harmonize with diabetes and kidney disease management.

Embracing a Vegan Lifestyle

Before we delve into the culinary delights that await, let us first explore the core tenets of veganism. A vegan lifestyle involves abstaining from the consumption of animal-derived products, which includes meat, dairy, eggs, and honey. It extends beyond dietary choices and encompasses a broader philosophy of compassion, environmental awareness, and ethical considerations.

By choosing a vegan diet, individuals reduce their carbon footprint, as animal agriculture is a significant contributor to greenhouse gas emissions. Moreover, adopting a plant-based diet promotes animal welfare by reducing the demand for animal products and supporting a more sustainable food system.

The Connection between Diabetes and Kidney Disease

Understanding the link between diabetes and kidney disease is essential in comprehending the rationale behind the recommended dietary choices. Diabetes is a metabolic disorder characterized by elevated blood sugar levels resulting from either insufficient insulin production or ineffective insulin utilization. Over time, chronically high blood sugar can damage various organs and systems within the body, including the kidneys.

Diabetic nephropathy, or kidney disease related to diabetes, is a common complication and a leading cause of end-stage renal disease (ESRD). The kidneys play a vital role in filtering waste products and excess fluids from the blood, maintaining a delicate balance of electrolytes and controlling blood pressure. The damage caused by uncontrolled diabetes compromises these functions, leading to the gradual decline of kidney function and necessitating stringent dietary management.

The Vegan Advantage for Diabetes and Kidney Health

The adoption of a vegan diet has garnered attention in recent years for its potential health benefits, particularly in managing chronic conditions such as diabetes and kidney disease. Various studies have highlighted the positive impact of plant-based nutrition in controlling blood sugar levels and mitigating the risk of developing kidney complications.

Plant-based diets are typically rich in fiber, antioxidants, and phytonutrients, which promote cardiovascular health and reduce inflammation—a crucial aspect in managing diabetes and kidney disease. The reduction of saturated fat and cholesterol inherent in a vegan diet may also contribute to improved blood lipid profiles and better glycemic control.

Nutritional Guidelines for Diabetes and Kidney Health

As we embark on this culinary journey, it is essential to establish a foundation of nutritional guidelines that will inform our recipe selections. The primary focus revolves around managing blood sugar levels and supporting kidney function through mindful dietary choices.

Carbohydrates: Carbohydrates play a significant role in blood glucose regulation, and selecting the right kind is essential for individuals with diabetes. Complex carbohydrates with a low glycemic index are preferable, as they result in slower and steadier increases in blood sugar levels. Whole grains, legumes, and non-starchy vegetables are excellent sources of complex carbohydrates.

Protein: Protein is a vital macronutrient necessary for tissue repair, enzyme production, and immune function. In the context of diabetes and kidney health, it is crucial to strike a balance between protein intake and kidney function. Plant-based protein sources such as tofu, tempeh, legumes, and quinoa offer healthy alternatives to animal-based proteins.

Fats: Dietary fats are a concentrated source of energy and play a role in absorbing fat-soluble vitamins. Opting for healthy fats, such as those found in avocados, nuts, seeds, and olive oil, can support heart health and contribute to overall well-being.

Sodium and Potassium: Sodium intake should be moderated to help manage blood pressure, especially in individuals with kidney disease. On the other hand, potassium-rich foods are beneficial for kidney health but may need to be limited in certain kidney conditions. Striking a balance between sodium and potassium intake is crucial in supporting kidney function.

Fluid Intake: For individuals with kidney disease, fluid intake may need to be adjusted based on their kidney function. Proper hydration is vital, but excessive fluid intake can strain the kidneys.

Tips for Meal Planning and Preparation

Embarking on a new culinary adventure requires thoughtful planning and preparation. As we progress through the chapters of this guide, we offer valuable tips to streamline your meal planning and ensure that you savor each recipe to the fullest.

Keep it Balanced: A balanced vegan diet is not only nutritionally sound but also enhances the overall dining experience. Include a diverse range of fruits, vegetables, whole grains, legumes, nuts, and seeds to meet your nutritional needs and elevate the flavors in your dishes.

Read Labels Mindfully: When opting for packaged ingredients, be mindful of the nutritional content, especially regarding sugar, sodium, and fat. Choose low-sodium or no-added-sugar versions to maintain better control over your dietary intake.

Experiment with Flavors and Textures: Embrace the vast palette of flavors and textures that plant-based ingredients offer. Incorporate fresh herbs, spices, and condiments to elevate the taste and appearance of your dishes, making each meal a delightful experience.

Batch Cooking and Freezing: Save time and effort by preparing larger quantities of certain dishes and freezing them for later consumption. This practice allows you to have ready-to-eat meals on hand during busy days, making it easier to adhere to your dietary goals.

Chapter 1: 30 Day Meal Plan

Week 1: Daily meal plan

Day 1:

Breakfast: Vegan Blueberry Chia Seed Pudding

Lunch: Lentil and Vegetable Soup

Dinner: Vegan Lentil Shepherd's Pie

Snack: Guacamole with Veggie Sticks

Dessert: Vegan Chocolate Avocado Mousse

Day 2:

Breakfast: Quinoa and Fruit Breakfast Bowl

Lunch: Vegan Chickpea Salad Sandwich

Dinner: Vegan Mushroom Stroganoff

Snack: Vegan Hummus with Pita Bread

Dessert: Vegan Banana Oat Cookies

Day 3:

Breakfast: Tofu Scramble with Spinach and Tomatoes

Lunch: Mediterranean Quinoa Salad

Dinner: Cauliflower and Chickpea Curry

Snack: Roasted Chickpeas with Spices

Dessert: Vegan Blueberry Lemon Bars

Day 4:

Breakfast: Oatmeal with Almond Milk and Berries

Lunch: Spicy Tofu and Vegetable Stir-Fry

Dinner: Vegan Ratatouille

Snack: Vegan Spinach and Artichoke Dip

Dessert: Chia Seed Chocolate Pudding

Day 5:

Breakfast: Vegan Banana Pancakes

Lunch: Vegan Cauliflower Fried Rice

Dinner: Quinoa Stuffed Portobello Mushrooms

Snack: Rice Paper Spring Rolls with Peanut Sauce

Dessert: Vegan Apple Crisp

Day 6:

Breakfast: Avocado Toast with Lime and Cilantro

Lunch: Zucchini Noodles with Pesto Sauce

Dinner: Vegan Butternut Squash Risotto

Snack: Vegan Stuffed Mushrooms

Dessert: Almond Butter Energy Bites

Day 7:

Breakfast: Sweet Potato and Black Bean Breakfast Burrito

Lunch: Black Bean and Sweet Potato Tacos

Dinner: Spicy Vegan Black Bean Enchiladas

Snack: Baked Sweet Potato Fries

Dessert: Vegan Raspberry Coconut Popsicles

Week 2: Daily meal plan

Day 8:

Breakfast: Vegan Breakfast Burrito Bowl

Lunch: Vegan Eggplant Parmesan

Dinner: Vegan Eggplant Lasagna

Snack: Vegan Buffalo Cauliflower Bites

Dessert: Vegan Carrot Cake Cupcakes

Day 9:

Breakfast: Mixed Berry Smoothie Bowl

Lunch: Vegan Buddha Bowl with Tahini Dressing

Dinner: Vegan Thai Green Curry

Snack: Cucumber Avocado Sushi Rolls

Dessert: Dairy-Free Chocolate Fudge

Day 10:

Breakfast: Vegan Breakfast Casserole with Hash Browns

Lunch: Vegan Stuffed Bell Peppers

Dinner: Vegan Baked Falafel with Lemon Tahini Sauce

Snack: Vegan Bruschetta with Tomato and Basil

Dessert: Vegan Mango Sorbet

Day 11:

Breakfast: Vegan Blueberry Chia Seed Pudding

Lunch: Lentil and Vegetable Soup

Dinner: Vegan Lentil Shepherd's Pie

Snack: Guacamole with Veggie Sticks

Dessert: Vegan Chocolate Avocado Mousse

Day 12:

Breakfast: Quinoa and Fruit Breakfast Bowl

Lunch: Vegan Chickpea Salad Sandwich

Dinner: Vegan Mushroom Stroganoff

Snack: Vegan Hummus with Pita Bread

Dessert: Vegan Banana Oat Cookies

Day 13:

Breakfast: Tofu Scramble with Spinach and Tomatoes

Lunch: Mediterranean Quinoa Salad

Dinner: Cauliflower and Chickpea Curry

Snack: Roasted Chickpeas with Spices

Dessert: Vegan Blueberry Lemon Bars

Day 14:

Breakfast: Oatmeal with Almond Milk and Berries

Lunch: Spicy Tofu and Vegetable Stir-Fry

Dinner: Vegan Ratatouille

Snack: Vegan Spinach and Artichoke Dip

Dessert: Chia Seed Chocolate Pudding

Week 3: Daily meal plan

Day 15:

Breakfast: Vegan Banana Pancakes

Lunch: Vegan Cauliflower Fried Rice

Dinner: Quinoa Stuffed Portobello Mushrooms

Snack: Rice Paper Spring Rolls with Peanut Sauce

Dessert: Vegan Apple Crisp

Day 16:

Breakfast: Avocado Toast with Lime and Cilantro

Lunch: Zucchini Noodles with Pesto Sauce

Dinner: Vegan Butternut Squash Risotto

Snack: Vegan Stuffed Mushrooms

Dessert: Almond Butter Energy Bites

Day 17:

Breakfast: Sweet Potato and Black Bean Breakfast Burrito

Lunch: Black Bean and Sweet Potato Tacos

Dinner: Spicy Vegan Black Bean Enchiladas

Snack: Baked Sweet Potato Fries

Dessert: Vegan Raspberry Coconut Popsicles

Day 18:

Breakfast: Vegan Breakfast Burrito Bowl

Lunch: Vegan Eggplant Parmesan

Dinner: Vegan Eggplant Lasagna

Snack: Vegan Buffalo Cauliflower Bites

Dessert: Vegan Carrot Cake Cupcakes

Day 19:

Breakfast: Mixed Berry Smoothie Bowl

Lunch: Vegan Buddha Bowl with Tahini Dressing

Dinner: Vegan Thai Green Curry

Snack: Cucumber Avocado Sushi Rolls

Dessert: Dairy-Free Chocolate Fudge

Day 20:

Breakfast: Vegan Breakfast Casserole with Hash Browns

Lunch: Vegan Stuffed Bell Peppers

Dinner: Vegan Baked Falafel with Lemon Tahini Sauce

Snack: Vegan Bruschetta with Tomato and Basil

Dessert: Vegan Mango Sorbet

Day 21:

Breakfast: Vegan Blueberry Chia Seed Pudding

Lunch: Lentil and Vegetable Soup

Dinner: Vegan Lentil Shepherd's Pie

Snack: Guacamole with Veggie Sticks

Dessert: Vegan Chocolate Avocado Mousse

Week 4: Daily meal plan

Day 22:

Breakfast: Quinoa and Fruit Breakfast Bowl

Lunch: Vegan Chickpea Salad Sandwich

Dinner: Vegan Mushroom Stroganoff

Snack: Vegan Hummus with Pita Bread

Dessert: Vegan Banana Oat Cookies

Day 23:

Breakfast: Tofu Scramble with Spinach and Tomatoes

Lunch: Mediterranean Quinoa Salad

Dinner: Cauliflower and Chickpea Curry

Snack: Roasted Chickpeas with Spices

Dessert: Vegan Blueberry Lemon Bars

Day 24:

Breakfast: Oatmeal with Almond Milk and Berries

Lunch: Spicy Tofu and Vegetable Stir-Fry

Dinner: Vegan Ratatouille

Snack: Vegan Spinach and Artichoke Dip

Dessert: Chia Seed Chocolate Pudding

Day 25:

Breakfast: Vegan Banana Pancakes

Lunch: Vegan Cauliflower Fried Rice

Dinner: Quinoa Stuffed Portobello Mushrooms

Snack: Rice Paper Spring Rolls with Peanut Sauce

Dessert: Vegan Apple Crisp

Day 26:

Breakfast: Avocado Toast with Lime and Cilantro

Lunch: Zucchini Noodles with Pesto Sauce

Dinner: Vegan Butternut Squash Risotto

Snack: Vegan Stuffed Mushrooms

Dessert: Almond Butter Energy Bites

Day 27:

Breakfast: Sweet Potato and Black Bean Breakfast Burrito

Lunch: Black Bean and Sweet Potato Tacos

Dinner: Spicy Vegan Black Bean Enchiladas

Snack: Baked Sweet Potato Fries

Dessert: Vegan Raspberry Coconut Popsicles

Day 28:

Breakfast: Vegan Breakfast Burrito Bowl

Lunch: Vegan Eggplant Parmesan

Dinner: Vegan Eggplant Lasagna

Snack: Vegan Buffalo Cauliflower Bites

Dessert: Vegan Carrot Cake Cupcakes

Day 29:

Breakfast: Mixed Berry Smoothie Bowl

Lunch: Vegan Buddha Bowl with Tahini Dressing

Dinner: Vegan Thai Green Curry

Snack: Cucumber Avocado Sushi Rolls

Dessert: Dairy-Free Chocolate Fudge

Day 30:

Breakfast: Vegan Breakfast Casserole with Hash Browns

Lunch: Vegan Stuffed Bell Peppers

Dinner: Vegan Baked Falafel with Lemon Tahini Sauce

Snack: Vegan Bruschetta with Tomato and Basil

Dessert: Vegan Mango Sorbet

Chapter 2: Breakfast Recipes

Breakfast is often hailed as the most important meal of the day, providing us with the energy and nutrients to kickstart our morning. For those looking for delicious and nutritious vegan options that cater to diabetes and kidney health, we present a delightful collection of breakfast recipes. These plant-based dishes are not only flavorful but also packed with essential vitamins and minerals to support your well-being. Let's dive into the kitchen and explore these scrumptious creations.

Vegan Blueberry Chia Seed Pudding

Ingredients:

- 1 cup unsweetened almond milk
- 3 tablespoons chia seeds
- 1 tablespoon maple syrup
- 1/2 teaspoon vanilla extract
- 1/2 cup fresh blueberries

Instructions:

1. In a bowl, combine almond milk, chia seeds, maple syrup, and vanilla extract.

2. Stir well and refrigerate the mixture overnight or for at least 4 hours to allow the chia seeds to expand and create a pudding-like texture.

3. Before serving, top the pudding with fresh blueberries for a burst of flavor and added antioxidants.

Quinoa and Fruit Breakfast Bowl

Ingredients:

- 1 cup cooked quinoa
- 1/2 cup sliced strawberries
- 1/2 cup diced mango
- 1/4 cup pomegranate arils
- 2 tablespoons chopped almonds
- 1 tablespoon agave syrup

Instructions:

1. Prepare the cooked quinoa according to package instructions and let it cool slightly.

2. In a serving bowl, combine the cooked quinoa, sliced strawberries, diced mango, and pomegranate arils.

3. Sprinkle chopped almonds on top for a delightful crunch and drizzle with agave syrup to enhance the sweetness.

Tofu Scramble with Spinach and Tomatoes

Ingredients:

- 1 block firm tofu, crumbled
- 1 cup fresh spinach leaves
- 1 cup cherry tomatoes, halved
- 1/2 teaspoon turmeric powder
- 1/2 teaspoon garlic powder
- 1/4 teaspoon ground cumin
- Salt and pepper to taste

Instructions:

1. Heat a non-stick skillet over medium heat and add the crumbled tofu, turmeric powder, garlic powder, and ground cumin.

2. Cook for about 5 minutes, stirring occasionally, until the tofu is lightly browned and seasoned.

3. Add fresh spinach leaves and halved cherry tomatoes to the skillet and continue cooking for an additional 3-4 minutes until the vegetables are tender.

4. Season with salt and pepper to taste, and serve this protein-packed scramble for a savory breakfast treat.

Oatmeal with Almond Milk and Berries

Ingredients:

- 1 cup rolled oats
- 2 cups unsweetened almond milk
- 1 cup mixed berries (blueberries, raspberries, strawberries)
- 1 tablespoon maple syrup

- 1 tablespoon almond butter

Instructions:

1. In a saucepan, combine rolled oats and almond milk. Bring to a simmer over medium heat, stirring occasionally.
2. Reduce heat to low and continue cooking for 5-7 minutes, or until the oats are tender and creamy.
3. Stir in mixed berries, maple syrup, and almond butter for added sweetness and flavor.
4. Serve this comforting bowl of oatmeal with a colorful medley of berries to start your day on a delightful note.

Vegan Banana Pancakes

Ingredients:

- 1 cup all-purpose flour
- 2 tablespoons coconut sugar
- 2 teaspoons baking powder
- 1/4 teaspoon salt
- 1 cup mashed ripe bananas (about 2 large bananas)
- 1 cup unsweetened almond milk

- 1 teaspoon vanilla extract

Instructions:

1. In a large mixing bowl, whisk together the all-purpose flour, coconut sugar, baking powder, and salt.
2. In a separate bowl, combine the mashed bananas, almond milk, and vanilla extract.
3. Gradually add the wet ingredients to the dry ingredients, stirring until just combined.
4. Heat a non-stick skillet over medium heat and lightly grease the surface with cooking spray or vegan butter.
5. Pour about 1/4 cup of pancake batter onto the skillet for each pancake. Cook until bubbles form on the surface, then flip and cook until golden brown on both sides.
6. Serve these fluffy vegan banana pancakes with a drizzle of maple syrup for a delightful breakfast treat.

Avocado Toast with Lime and Cilantro

Ingredients:

- 2 slices whole-grain bread, toasted
- 1 ripe avocado
- Juice of half a lime
- Fresh cilantro leaves
- Salt and pepper to taste

Instructions:

1. Scoop out the flesh of the ripe avocado into a bowl and mash it with a fork until smooth.
2. Add lime juice, fresh cilantro leaves, salt, and pepper to the mashed avocado and mix well.
3. Spread the avocado mixture onto the toasted whole-grain bread slices.
4. Garnish with additional cilantro leaves for a burst of freshness and enjoy this simple yet satisfying avocado toast.

Sweet Potato and Black Bean Breakfast Burrito

Ingredients:

- 2 large whole-grain tortillas
- 1 cup cooked and mashed sweet potatoes
- 1 cup black beans, rinsed and drained
- 1/2 cup diced red bell pepper
- 1/4 cup diced red onion
- 1/4 teaspoon chili powder
- 1/4 teaspoon cumin
- Salt and pepper to taste

Instructions:

1. In a large skillet, sauté diced red bell pepper and red onion until softened.
2. Add cooked and mashed sweet potatoes, black beans, chili powder, cumin, salt, and pepper. Stir until well combined and heated through.
3. Warm the whole-grain tortillas, then spoon the sweet potato and black bean mixture onto each tortilla.

4. Roll the tortillas into burritos and serve this flavorful and filling breakfast option.

Vegan Breakfast Burrito Bowl

Ingredients:

- 1 cup cooked brown rice
- 1 cup black beans, rinsed and drained
- 1 cup diced avocado
- 1/2 cup diced tomatoes
- 1/4 cup diced red onion
- 2 tablespoons chopped fresh cilantro
- 1 tablespoon lime juice
- Salt and pepper to taste

Instructions:

1. In a serving bowl, arrange cooked brown rice as the base of the burrito bowl.
2. Top with black beans, diced avocado, diced tomatoes, and diced red onion.
3. Drizzle lime juice over the bowl and season with salt and pepper.

4. Garnish with chopped fresh cilantro for a burst of color and flavor in this satisfying breakfast bowl.

Mixed Berry Smoothie Bowl

Ingredients:

- 1 cup frozen mixed berries (blueberries, raspberries, strawberries)
- 1 ripe banana
- 1/2 cup unsweetened almond milk
- 1 tablespoon chia seeds
- Toppings: fresh berries, sliced banana, granola, shredded coconut

Instructions:

1. In a blender, combine frozen mixed berries, ripe banana, almond milk, and chia seeds.
2. Blend until smooth and creamy, adding more almond milk if needed to reach the desired consistency.
3. Pour the smoothie into a bowl and arrange fresh berries, sliced banana, granola, and shredded coconut on top.

4. Savor this refreshing and nutrient-packed mixed berry smoothie bowl to brighten up your morning.

Vegan Breakfast Casserole with Hash Browns

Ingredients:

- 4 cups frozen hash browns
- 1 cup diced bell peppers (assorted colors)
- 1 cup diced zucchini
- 1 cup chopped kale leaves
- 1 cup sliced cherry tomatoes
- 1 block firm tofu, crumbled
- 1/2 cup unsweetened almond milk
- 2 tablespoons nutritional yeast
- 1 teaspoon garlic powder
- 1/2 teaspoon turmeric powder
- Salt and pepper to taste

Instructions:

1. Preheat the oven to 375°F (190°C) and lightly grease a casserole dish.

2. In a large bowl, combine frozen hash browns, diced bell peppers, diced zucchini, chopped kale leaves, and sliced cherry tomatoes.

3. In a separate bowl, mix crumbled firm tofu, almond milk, nutritional yeast, garlic powder, turmeric powder, salt, and pepper to create a savory tofu mixture.

4. Spread half of the hash brown and vegetable mixture into the casserole dish, then pour half of the tofu mixture over it. Repeat with the remaining ingredients.

5. Bake the breakfast casserole for 30-35 minutes or until the top is golden and the casserole is heated through.

6. Allow the casserole to cool slightly before serving this hearty and nutritious breakfast dish.

Chapter 3: Lunch Recipes

Lunchtime offers a delightful opportunity to indulge in healthy and flavorful vegan dishes that satisfy both your taste buds and nutritional needs. In this chapter, we present delectable and easy-to-prepare lunch recipes that are perfect for those managing diabetes and kidney disease. These dishes are not only packed with essential nutrients but also designed to appeal to your palate.

Lentil and Vegetable Soup

Ingredients:

- 1 cup green lentils, rinsed and drained
- 4 cups vegetable broth
- 1 medium onion, finely chopped
- 2 cloves garlic, minced
- 2 carrots, diced
- 2 celery stalks, diced
- 1 cup diced tomatoes (canned or fresh)
- 1 teaspoon ground cumin
- 1 teaspoon paprika

- 1/2 teaspoon dried thyme
- Salt and pepper to taste
- Fresh parsley for garnish

Instructions:

1. In a large pot, sauté the onions and garlic with a splash of vegetable broth until translucent.
2. Add the diced carrots and celery, and continue to cook for a few minutes until slightly softened.
3. Stir in the lentils, vegetable broth, diced tomatoes, cumin, paprika, and dried thyme.
4. Bring the mixture to a boil, then reduce the heat and let it simmer for about 20-25 minutes or until the lentils are tender.
5. Season with salt and pepper to taste.
6. Serve hot, garnished with fresh parsley.

Vegan Chickpea Salad Sandwich

Ingredients:

- 1 can (15 oz) chickpeas, drained and rinsed
- 1/4 cup vegan mayonnaise
- 1 tablespoon Dijon mustard

- 1 celery stalk, finely chopped
- 1/4 cup red bell pepper, diced
- 2 tablespoons red onion, finely chopped
- 1 tablespoon fresh lemon juice
- 1/2 teaspoon ground cumin
- Salt and pepper to taste
- Whole grain bread or pita pockets
- Lettuce leaves and sliced tomatoes for serving

Instructions:

1. In a medium bowl, mash the chickpeas with a fork until partly crushed.
2. Add the vegan mayonnaise, Dijon mustard, chopped celery, diced red bell pepper, red onion, fresh lemon juice, ground cumin, salt, and pepper. Mix well to combine.
3. Adjust seasonings to taste.
4. Spread the chickpea salad on whole grain bread or stuff it into pita pockets.
5. Top with lettuce leaves and sliced tomatoes.
6. Serve as a satisfying sandwich for lunch.

Mediterranean Quinoa Salad

Ingredients:

- 1 cup cooked quinoa
- 1 cup cucumber, diced
- 1 cup cherry tomatoes, halved
- 1/2 cup Kalamata olives, pitted and sliced
- 1/4 cup red onion, finely chopped
- 1/4 cup fresh parsley, chopped
- 1/4 cup fresh mint leaves, chopped
- 1/4 cup extra-virgin olive oil
- 2 tablespoons lemon juice
- 1 clove garlic, minced
- Salt and pepper to taste
- Vegan feta cheese, crumbled (optional)

Instructions:

1. In a large bowl, combine the cooked quinoa, diced cucumber, halved cherry tomatoes, sliced Kalamata olives, chopped red onion, chopped parsley, and chopped mint leaves.

2. In a separate small bowl, whisk together the extra-virgin olive oil, lemon juice, minced garlic, salt, and pepper to make the dressing.

3. Pour the dressing over the quinoa mixture and toss well to coat.

4. If desired, sprinkle crumbled vegan feta cheese on top for added creaminess and flavor.

5. Chill the salad in the refrigerator for at least 30 minutes before serving.

Spicy Tofu and Vegetable Stir-Fry

Ingredients:

- 1 block firm tofu, drained and cubed
- 2 tablespoons soy sauce (or tamari for a gluten-free option)
- 1 tablespoon cornstarch
- 1 tablespoon vegetable oil
- 1 red bell pepper, sliced
- 1 yellow bell pepper, sliced
- 1 cup broccoli florets
- 1 cup snap peas
- 2 cloves garlic, minced

- 1 tablespoon fresh ginger, grated
- 2 tablespoons sriracha sauce (adjust to your spice preference)
- 2 tablespoons hoisin sauce
- 1 tablespoon rice vinegar
- 2 green onions, chopped (green parts only)
- Sesame seeds for garnish

Instructions:

1. In a bowl, combine the cubed tofu with soy sauce and cornstarch, ensuring all pieces are coated.
2. In a large skillet or wok, heat the vegetable oil over medium-high heat.
3. Add the marinated tofu and cook until it becomes golden and crispy on all sides. Remove the tofu from the skillet and set it aside.
4. In the same skillet, add the sliced red and yellow bell peppers, broccoli florets, and snap peas. Stir-fry for a few minutes until the vegetables are tender-crisp.
5. Add the minced garlic and grated ginger, and sauté for an additional minute.

6. Return the tofu to the skillet and mix well with the vegetables.

7. In a small bowl, whisk together the sriracha sauce, hoisin sauce, and rice vinegar to make the spicy sauce.

8. Pour the sauce over the tofu and vegetables, tossing everything to coat evenly.

9. Sprinkle chopped green onions and sesame seeds on top for garnish.

10. Serve the spicy tofu and vegetable stir-fry over cooked quinoa or brown rice.

Vegan Cauliflower Fried Rice

Ingredients:

- 1 medium cauliflower head, florets separated
- 2 tablespoons vegetable oil
- 1 cup frozen mixed vegetables (peas, carrots, corn, etc.)
- 2 cloves garlic, minced
- 2 tablespoons soy sauce (or tamari for a gluten-free option)
- 1 tablespoon sesame oil

- 2 green onions, chopped
- Sesame seeds for garnish

Instructions:

1. In a food processor, pulse the cauliflower florets until they resemble rice-like grains. Be careful not to overprocess, or it will turn into mush.
2. In a large skillet or wok, heat the vegetable oil over medium-high heat.
3. Add the frozen mixed vegetables and minced garlic, sautéing until the vegetables are heated through and tender.
4. Push the vegetables to one side of the skillet and add the cauliflower rice to the other side.
5. Drizzle the soy sauce and sesame oil over the cauliflower rice and toss everything together until well combined.
6. Cook for a few minutes, stirring occasionally, until the cauliflower rice is cooked but not mushy.
7. Garnish with chopped green onions and sesame seeds before serving.

Zucchini Noodles with Pesto Sauce

Ingredients:

- 4 medium zucchinis, spiralized into noodles
- 1 cup fresh basil leaves
- 1/4 cup pine nuts
- 2 cloves garlic, minced
- 1/4 cup nutritional yeast
- 1/4 cup extra-virgin olive oil
- 1 tablespoon lemon juice
- Salt and pepper to taste
- Cherry tomatoes for garnish

Instructions:

1. In a food processor, combine the fresh basil leaves, pine nuts, minced garlic, nutritional yeast, extra-virgin olive oil, and lemon juice. Blend until a smooth and creamy pesto sauce forms.

2. In a large pan, sauté the zucchini noodles with a little vegetable broth over medium heat until they soften slightly. Be careful not to overcook, as they should retain some crunch.

3. Add the prepared pesto sauce to the pan with the zucchini noodles, tossing well to coat evenly.

4. Season with salt and pepper to taste.

5. Garnish with halved cherry tomatoes before serving.

Black Bean and Sweet Potato Tacos

Ingredients:

- 1 can (15 oz) black beans, drained and rinsed
- 2 medium sweet potatoes, peeled and diced
- 1 tablespoon vegetable oil
- 1 teaspoon ground cumin
- 1 teaspoon chili powder
- 1/2 teaspoon smoked paprika
- Salt and pepper to taste
- Corn tortillas
- Avocado slices, diced red onion, and fresh cilantro for serving

Instructions:

1. In a large skillet, heat the vegetable oil over medium heat.

2. Add the diced sweet potatoes and sauté until they become tender and slightly crispy.

3. Stir in the drained black beans, ground cumin, chili powder, smoked paprika, salt, and pepper. Cook for a few more minutes to blend the flavors.

4. Warm the corn tortillas in a separate pan or microwave.

5. Assemble the tacos by filling each tortilla with the black bean and sweet potato mixture.

6. Top with avocado slices, diced red onion, and fresh cilantro for a burst of freshness and color.

7. Serve the tasty black bean and sweet potato tacos for a delightful lunch.

Vegan Eggplant Parmesan

Ingredients:

- 1 large eggplant, sliced into rounds
- 1 cup breadcrumbs (gluten-free if preferred)
- 1/2 cup nutritional yeast
- 1 teaspoon dried oregano
- 1 teaspoon dried basil
- 1/2 teaspoon garlic powder

- Salt and pepper to taste
- 1 cup marinara sauce (store-bought or homemade)
- Vegan mozzarella cheese (optional)
- Fresh basil leaves for garnish

Instructions:

1. Preheat the oven to 375°F (190°C).
2. In a shallow dish, mix together the breadcrumbs, nutritional yeast, dried oregano, dried basil, garlic powder, salt, and pepper to create the breading mixture.
3. Dip each eggplant slice into the breading mixture, ensuring both sides are coated evenly.
4. Place the breaded eggplant slices on a baking sheet lined with parchment paper.
5. Bake the eggplant in the preheated oven for about 20-25 minutes or until they become crispy and golden brown.
6. In a separate saucepan, warm the marinara sauce over medium heat.

7. Remove the baked eggplant slices from the oven and top each one with a spoonful of warm marinara sauce.

8. If desired, sprinkle vegan mozzarella cheese on top of each slice.

9. Return the eggplant slices to the oven and broil for a few minutes until the cheese melts and bubbles.

10. Garnish with fresh basil leaves before serving the mouthwatering vegan eggplant Parmesan.

Vegan Buddha Bowl with Tahini Dressing

Ingredients:

- 1 cup cooked quinoa
- 1 cup cooked chickpeas (canned or cooked from dried)
- 1 cup steamed broccoli florets
- 1 cup shredded carrots
- 1 cup sliced cucumber
- 1 avocado, sliced
- 1 tablespoon sesame seeds

- Fresh cilantro for garnish

Tahini Dressing:
- 1/4 cup tahini
- 2 tablespoons lemon juice
- 2 tablespoons water
- 1 tablespoon maple syrup
- 1 clove garlic, minced
- Salt and pepper to taste

Instructions:

1. In a large bowl, assemble the vegan Buddha bowl by arranging cooked quinoa, chickpeas, steamed broccoli florets, shredded carrots, sliced cucumber, and avocado.

2. Sprinkle sesame seeds on top for added texture and nuttiness.

3. For the tahini dressing, whisk together the tahini, lemon juice, water, maple syrup, minced garlic, salt, and pepper in a small bowl until smooth and creamy.

4. Drizzle the tahini dressing over the Buddha bowl or serve it on the side.

5. Garnish with fresh cilantro before enjoying the wholesome and vibrant flavors of this vegan Buddha bowl.

Vegan Stuffed Bell Peppers

Ingredients:

- 4 large bell peppers (any color)
- 1 cup cooked quinoa
- 1 cup cooked black beans (canned or cooked from dried)
- 1 cup diced tomatoes (canned or fresh)
- 1/2 cup corn kernels (frozen or fresh)
- 1/2 cup diced red onion
- 1/2 cup diced zucchini
- 1 clove garlic, minced
- 1 teaspoon ground cumin
- 1 teaspoon chili powder
- 1/2 teaspoon paprika
- Salt and pepper to taste
- Vegan cheese shreds (optional)

Instructions:

1. Preheat the oven to 375°F (190°C).
2. Cut off the tops of the bell peppers and remove the seeds and membranes from the inside.
3. In a large skillet, sauté the diced red onion and minced garlic with a splash of vegetable broth until softened.
4. Add the cooked quinoa, black beans, diced tomatoes, corn kernels, diced zucchini, ground cumin, chili powder, paprika, salt, and pepper. Mix well and cook for a few minutes to combine the flavors.
5. Stuff each bell pepper with the quinoa and vegetable mixture until they are generously filled.
6. Place the stuffed bell peppers in a baking dish and cover the dish with foil.
7. Bake the stuffed bell peppers in the preheated oven for about 25-30 minutes or until the peppers are tender.
8. If desired, sprinkle vegan cheese shreds on top of each stuffed pepper and return them to the oven, baking until the cheese melts and becomes gooey.

9. Serve the delightful vegan stuffed bell peppers as a hearty and wholesome lunch option.

Chapter 4: Dinner Recipes

In this chapter, we'll explore a delightful array of dinner recipes that are not only delectable but also fully vegan. These recipes are carefully crafted to cater to those with diabetes and kidney disease, focusing on ingredients that promote health and wellness. So, let's embark on a culinary adventure and prepare these wholesome dishes together.

Vegan Lentil Shepherd's Pie

Ingredients:

- 1 cup dried green lentils
- 3 cups vegetable broth
- 1 large onion, diced
- 2 cloves garlic, minced
- 2 carrots, diced
- 1 cup frozen peas
- 1 cup frozen corn
- 3 tablespoons tomato paste
- 1 tablespoon soy sauce
- 1 teaspoon dried thyme

- 1 teaspoon dried rosemary
- 4 cups mashed potatoes (made with plant-based milk and vegan butter)
- Salt and pepper to taste

Instructions:

1. In a large pot, combine the lentils and vegetable broth. Bring to a boil, then reduce heat and simmer for about 20 minutes or until the lentils are tender.
2. In a separate pan, sauté the onion and garlic until they become translucent. Add the carrots and cook for a few minutes until slightly softened.
3. Add the cooked lentils, frozen peas, frozen corn, tomato paste, soy sauce, dried thyme, and dried rosemary to the sautéed vegetables. Mix well and let it simmer for 5-10 minutes until the flavors meld.
4. Preheat the oven to 375°F (190°C). Transfer the lentil mixture to a baking dish and spread the mashed potatoes evenly over the top.
5. Bake in the preheated oven for 25-30 minutes or until the mashed potatoes develop a golden crust.

Serve hot and enjoy the comforting goodness of Vegan Lentil Shepherd's Pie.

Vegan Mushroom Stroganoff

Ingredients:

- 12 ounces (340g) white mushrooms, sliced
- 1 tablespoon olive oil
- 1 large onion, finely chopped
- 2 cloves garlic, minced
- 2 cups vegetable broth
- 1 tablespoon soy sauce
- 1 tablespoon Dijon mustard
- 1 cup plant-based sour cream
- 1 tablespoon flour (gluten-free if needed)
- Salt and pepper to taste
- Fresh parsley for garnish
- Cooked pasta or rice for serving

Instructions:

1. In a large skillet, heat the olive oil over medium heat. Add the chopped onion and garlic, sautéing until they turn soft and fragrant.

2. Add the sliced mushrooms to the skillet and cook until they release their moisture and become tender.

3. Stir in the vegetable broth, soy sauce, and Dijon mustard. Let the mixture simmer for a few minutes.

4. In a small bowl, whisk the plant-based sour cream and flour until smooth. Add the mixture to the skillet and stir well, allowing the sauce to thicken.

5. Season with salt and pepper to taste. Serve the Vegan Mushroom Stroganoff over cooked pasta or rice and garnish with fresh parsley.

Cauliflower and Chickpea Curry

Ingredients:

- 1 large cauliflower, cut into florets
- 1 can (15 ounces) chickpeas, drained and rinsed
- 1 tablespoon coconut oil
- 1 large onion, finely chopped
- 2 cloves garlic, minced
- 1 tablespoon grated ginger
- 1 can (14 ounces) coconut milk
- 2 tablespoons red curry paste
- 1 tablespoon curry powder

- 1 teaspoon turmeric powder
- 1 teaspoon cumin
- Salt and pepper to taste
- Fresh cilantro for garnish
- Cooked basmati rice for serving

Instructions:

1. In a large pot, heat the coconut oil over medium heat. Add the chopped onion, garlic, and grated ginger, sautéing until fragrant.
2. Stir in the red curry paste, curry powder, turmeric, and cumin. Cook for a minute or two to release the spices' aroma.
3. Add the cauliflower florets and chickpeas to the pot, mixing them well with the spices and onion mixture.
4. Pour in the coconut milk and bring the curry to a gentle boil. Reduce heat, cover, and let it simmer for about 15-20 minutes or until the cauliflower becomes tender.

5. Season with salt and pepper to taste. Serve the Cauliflower and Chickpea Curry over cooked basmati rice and garnish with fresh cilantro.

Vegan Ratatouille

Ingredients:

- 1 large eggplant, diced
- 1 zucchini, diced
- 1 yellow squash, diced
- 1 red bell pepper, diced
- 1 yellow bell pepper, diced
- 1 can (14 ounces) diced tomatoes
- 3 tablespoons olive oil
- 3 cloves garlic, minced
- 1 tablespoon tomato paste
- 1 teaspoon dried thyme
- 1 teaspoon dried oregano
- Salt and pepper to taste
- Fresh basil for garnish

Instructions:

1. Preheat the oven to 375°F (190°C). Place the diced eggplant, zucchini, yellow squash, red bell pepper, and yellow bell pepper on a baking sheet.

2. Drizzle with olive oil, making sure the vegetables are coated evenly. Season with salt and pepper, then toss to combine.

3. Roast the vegetables in the preheated oven for 20-25 minutes or until they become tender and slightly browned.

4. In a large skillet, heat the remaining olive oil over medium heat. Add the minced garlic and cook until fragrant.

5. Stir in the tomato paste, dried thyme, and dried oregano. Cook for a minute or two to infuse the flavors.

6. Add the diced tomatoes to the skillet and let it simmer for a few minutes.

7. Gently fold in the roasted vegetables, ensuring they are coated with the tomato sauce. Adjust the seasoning with salt and pepper if needed.

8. Serve the Vegan Ratatouille hot, garnished with fresh basil leaves.

Quinoa Stuffed Portobello Mushrooms

Ingredients:

- 4 large Portobello mushrooms
- 1 cup quinoa, rinsed and drained
- 2 cups vegetable broth
- 1 tablespoon olive oil
- 1 small onion, finely chopped
- 2 cloves garlic, minced
- 1 cup diced tomatoes
- 1 cup baby spinach, chopped
- 1/4 cup chopped fresh parsley
- 1/4 cup chopped walnuts
- Salt and pepper to taste
- Vegan shredded cheese (optional) for topping

Instructions:

1. Preheat the oven to 375°F (190°C). Remove the stems from the Portobello mushrooms and gently scrape out the gills to create more space for the filling.

2. In a medium saucepan, bring the vegetable broth to a boil. Add the rinsed quinoa and reduce heat to a simmer. Cover and cook for 15-20 minutes or until the quinoa is cooked and the liquid is absorbed.

3. In a separate skillet, heat the olive oil over medium heat. Add the chopped onion and garlic, sautéing until softened.

4. Stir in the diced tomatoes, baby spinach, chopped parsley, and chopped walnuts. Cook for a few minutes until the spinach wilts and the flavors meld.

5. Combine the cooked quinoa with the vegetable mixture and season with salt and pepper to taste.

6. Stuff each Portobello mushroom with the quinoa filling, pressing it down slightly to fit more.

7. Optional: Top the stuffed mushrooms with vegan shredded cheese for an extra layer of deliciousness.

8. Place the stuffed mushrooms on a baking sheet and bake in the preheated oven for 20-25 minutes or until the mushrooms are tender and the filling is heated through.

Vegan Butternut Squash Risotto

Ingredients:

- 2 cups cubed butternut squash
- 2 tablespoons olive oil
- 1 small onion, finely chopped
- 2 cloves garlic, minced
- 1 1/2 cups Arborio rice
- 1/2 cup dry white wine
- 4 cups vegetable broth
- 1 cup plant-based milk (such as almond or soy milk)
- 1/4 cup nutritional yeast
- 1 teaspoon dried thyme
- Salt and pepper to taste
- Fresh sage for garnish

Instructions:

1. Preheat the oven to 400°F (200°C). Toss the cubed butternut squash with 1 tablespoon of olive oil and season with salt and pepper. Roast the squash on a baking sheet for 20-25 minutes or until tender and slightly caramelized.

2. In a large saucepan, heat the remaining olive oil over medium heat. Add the chopped onion and garlic, sautéing until translucent.

3. Stir in the Arborio rice and cook for a minute or two until the rice is lightly toasted.

4. Pour in the dry white wine and let it simmer until most of the liquid is absorbed.

5. Gradually add the vegetable broth, one cup at a time, stirring constantly and allowing the liquid to be absorbed before adding more.

6. After about 15 minutes, when the rice is nearly tender, stir in the roasted butternut squash, plant-based milk, nutritional yeast, and dried thyme.

7. Continue to cook and stir until the rice reaches a creamy consistency and is fully cooked.

8. Season with salt and pepper to taste. Serve the Vegan Butternut Squash Risotto hot, garnished with fresh sage leaves.

Spicy Vegan Black Bean Enchiladas

Ingredients:

- 2 cups cooked black beans

- 1 tablespoon olive oil
- 1 small onion, finely chopped
- 2 cloves garlic, minced
- 1 can (14 ounces) diced tomatoes with green chilies
- 1 tablespoon chili powder
- 1 teaspoon cumin
- 1 teaspoon paprika
- Salt and pepper to taste
- 8-10 corn tortillas
- 1 cup enchilada sauce (store-bought or homemade)
- Vegan shredded cheese (optional) for topping
- Fresh cilantro and sliced jalapeños for garnish

Instructions:

1. Preheat the oven to 375°F (190°C). In a large skillet, heat the olive oil over medium heat. Add the chopped onion and garlic, sautéing until fragrant.
2. Stir in the cooked black beans, diced tomatoes with green chilies, chili powder, cumin, and paprika. Cook for a few minutes to allow the flavors to meld. Season with salt and pepper to taste.

3. In a separate skillet, warm the corn tortillas for a few seconds on each side until they become pliable.

4. Spoon the black bean mixture onto each corn tortilla and roll it up tightly, placing the enchiladas seam side down in a baking dish.

5. Pour the enchilada sauce over the rolled tortillas, making sure they are well coated.

6. Optional: Sprinkle vegan shredded cheese on top of the enchiladas for an extra layer of gooey goodness.

7. Bake the Spicy Vegan Black Bean Enchiladas in the preheated oven for 20-25 minutes or until they are heated through and the sauce is bubbly.

8. Garnish with fresh cilantro and sliced jalapeños before serving.

Vegan Eggplant Lasagna

Ingredients:

- 1 large eggplant, thinly sliced lengthwise
- 2 tablespoons olive oil
- 1 small onion, finely chopped
- 2 cloves garlic, minced
- 1 can (14 ounces) crushed tomatoes

- 1 can (14 ounces) tomato sauce
- 1 tablespoon tomato paste
- 1 teaspoon dried oregano
- 1 teaspoon dried basil
- Salt and pepper to taste
- 2 cups plant-based ricotta cheese
- 1/4 cup nutritional yeast
- 2 cups vegan shredded mozzarella cheese
- Fresh basil for garnish

Instructions:

1. Preheat the oven to 375°F (190°C). On a baking sheet, arrange the eggplant slices and brush them with olive oil. Season with salt and pepper.

2. Roast the eggplant in the preheated oven for 15-20 minutes or until they become tender and slightly browned. Remove from the oven and set aside.

3. In a large skillet, heat the olive oil over medium heat. Add the chopped onion and garlic, sautéing until softened and fragrant.

4. Stir in the crushed tomatoes, tomato sauce, tomato paste, dried oregano, and dried basil. Let the sauce

simmer for a few minutes to blend the flavors. Season with salt and pepper to taste.

5. In a separate bowl, combine the plant-based ricotta cheese and nutritional yeast. Mix well until smooth and creamy.

6. To assemble the lasagna, spread a layer of the tomato sauce on the bottom of a baking dish. Add a layer of roasted eggplant slices, followed by a layer of the ricotta mixture and vegan shredded mozzarella cheese.

7. Repeat the layers until all the ingredients are used, finishing with a layer of tomato sauce and vegan shredded mozzarella cheese on top.

8. Bake the Vegan Eggplant Lasagna in the preheated oven for 25-30 minutes or until the cheese is melted and bubbly.

9. Garnish with fresh basil before serving.

Vegan Thai Green Curry

Ingredients:

- 1 tablespoon coconut oil
- 1 small onion, finely chopped

- 2 cloves garlic, minced
- 1 tablespoon grated ginger
- 2 tablespoons Thai green curry paste
- 1 can (14 ounces) coconut milk
- 1 cup vegetable broth
- 2 tablespoons soy sauce
- 1 tablespoon brown sugar
- 1 cup sliced bell peppers (a mix of red, green, and yellow)
- 1 cup sliced carrots
- 1 cup sliced zucchini
- 1 cup sliced bamboo shoots (optional)
- 1 cup baby corn (optional)
- 1 cup fresh basil leaves
- Cooked jasmine rice for serving

Instructions:

1. In a large wok or skillet, heat the coconut oil over medium heat. Add the chopped onion, garlic, and grated ginger, sautéing until fragrant.
2. Stir in the Thai green curry paste and cook for a minute or two to release its flavors.

3. Pour in the coconut milk, vegetable broth, soy sauce, and brown sugar. Bring the mixture to a gentle boil.

4. Add the sliced bell peppers, carrots, zucchini, bamboo shoots, and baby corn (if using). Let the curry simmer for about 10-15 minutes or until the vegetables become tender.

5. Fold in the fresh basil leaves and cook for an additional minute to infuse the curry with their aroma.

6. Serve the Vegan Thai Green Curry hot over cooked jasmine rice.

Vegan Baked Falafel with Lemon Tahini Sauce

Ingredients for Falafel:

- 2 cups cooked or canned chickpeas, drained and rinsed
- 1 small onion, finely chopped
- 3 cloves garlic, minced
- 1 cup fresh parsley leaves

- 1 teaspoon ground cumin

- 1 teaspoon ground coriander

- 1/2 teaspoon baking soda

- 2 tablespoons chickpea flour (or all-purpose flour)

- Salt and pepper to taste

- Olive oil for brushing

Ingredients for Lemon Tahini Sauce:
- 1/2 cup tahini

- 1/4 cup water

- Juice of 1 lemon

- 2 cloves garlic, minced

- Salt to taste

Instructions for Falafel:
1. Preheat the oven to 375°F (190°C). In a food processor, combine the chickpeas, chopped onion, minced garlic, fresh parsley, ground cumin, ground coriander, baking soda, chickpea flour, salt, and pepper.

2. Pulse the mixture until well combined, but not completely smooth (some texture is desired).

3. Form the falafel mixture into small patties or balls and place them on a baking sheet lined with parchment paper.

4. Brush the falafel with olive oil and bake in the preheated oven for 20-25 minutes or until they become golden and crispy.

Instructions for Lemon Tahini Sauce:

1. In a small bowl, whisk together the tahini, water, lemon juice, minced garlic, and salt until the sauce reaches a smooth and creamy consistency.

To Serve:

Serve the Vegan Baked Falafel hot, drizzled with Lemon Tahini Sauce and garnished with fresh parsley and a sprinkle of paprika for an extra burst of color and flavor.

Chapter 5: Snacks and Appetizers

These delectable vegan snacks and appetizers are sure to be a hit with your family and friends. They offer a variety of flavors and textures, making them suitable for any occasion. Enjoy these delicious plant-based treats and savor the health benefits they provide. Whether you're hosting a party or simply enjoying a relaxing evening at home, these recipes will add a burst of flavor and nutrition to your table. Happy cooking!

Guacamole with Veggie Sticks

Ingredients:

- 3 ripe avocados
- 1 small onion, finely diced
- 2 cloves of garlic, minced
- 1 jalapeno pepper, seeds removed and finely chopped
- 2 ripe tomatoes, diced
- 1 lime, juiced
- Salt and pepper to taste

- Fresh cilantro leaves, chopped
- Assorted veggie sticks (carrots, celery, bell peppers) for serving

Instructions:

1. Cut the avocados in half, remove the pits, and scoop the flesh into a mixing bowl.
2. Mash the avocado with a fork until it reaches your desired consistency (chunky or smooth).
3. Add the diced onion, minced garlic, and chopped jalapeno pepper to the bowl. Mix well.
4. Gently fold in the diced tomatoes and lime juice into the avocado mixture.
5. Season with salt and pepper to taste.
6. Garnish the guacamole with freshly chopped cilantro leaves.
7. Serve the guacamole with a platter of assorted veggie sticks for dipping.

Vegan Hummus with Pita Bread

Ingredients:

- 1 can (15 oz) chickpeas, drained and rinsed

- 3 tablespoons tahini
- 3 tablespoons lemon juice
- 2 cloves of garlic
- 2 tablespoons olive oil
- 1/2 teaspoon ground cumin
- Salt to taste
- Water (as needed for desired consistency)
- Pita bread, cut into triangles, for serving

Instructions:

1. In a food processor, combine the chickpeas, tahini, lemon juice, garlic, olive oil, and ground cumin.
2. Blend the ingredients until smooth, adding water gradually as needed for your desired hummus consistency.
3. Season the hummus with salt to taste and blend again to incorporate the seasoning.
4. Transfer the hummus to a serving bowl and drizzle with a little olive oil for extra flavor.
5. Serve the vegan hummus with pita bread triangles for dipping.

Roasted Chickpeas with Spices

Ingredients:

- 1 can (15 oz) chickpeas, drained and rinsed
- 2 tablespoons olive oil
- 1 teaspoon ground cumin
- 1/2 teaspoon smoked paprika
- 1/2 teaspoon garlic powder
- Salt and pepper to taste

Instructions:

1. Preheat the oven to 400°F (200°C) and line a baking sheet with parchment paper.
2. In a bowl, toss the chickpeas with olive oil, ground cumin, smoked paprika, garlic powder, salt, and pepper until evenly coated.
3. Spread the seasoned chickpeas in a single layer on the prepared baking sheet.
4. Roast the chickpeas in the preheated oven for 25-30 minutes, or until they become crispy and golden brown.
5. Remove the roasted chickpeas from the oven and let them cool slightly before serving.

Vegan Spinach and Artichoke Dip

Ingredients:

- 2 cups fresh baby spinach, chopped
- 1 can (14 oz) artichoke hearts, drained and chopped
- 1 cup vegan cream cheese
- 1/2 cup vegan mayonnaise
- 1/2 cup vegan sour cream
- 1/2 cup nutritional yeast
- 1 teaspoon garlic powder
- 1/2 teaspoon onion powder
- Salt and pepper to taste
- Tortilla chips or pita bread, for serving

Instructions:

1. Preheat the oven to 375°F (190°C) and lightly grease a baking dish.
2. In a large mixing bowl, combine the chopped spinach, chopped artichoke hearts, vegan cream cheese, vegan mayonnaise, vegan sour cream, and nutritional yeast.
3. Stir in the garlic powder, onion powder, salt, and pepper until well combined.

4. Transfer the mixture to the prepared baking dish and spread it evenly.

5. Bake in the preheated oven for 20-25 minutes or until the dip is heated through and slightly bubbly.

6. Serve the vegan spinach and artichoke dip with tortilla chips or pita bread.

Rice Paper Spring Rolls with Peanut Sauce

Ingredients for Spring Rolls:

- 10 rice paper wrappers
- 1 cup cooked rice vermicelli noodles
- 1 cup shredded lettuce
- 1 cup julienned carrots
- 1 cup julienned cucumber
- 1/2 cup fresh mint leaves
- 1/2 cup fresh cilantro leaves
- 1/2 cup julienned red bell pepper
- 1/2 cup julienned mango (optional)

Ingredients for Peanut Sauce:

- 1/4 cup creamy peanut butter
- 2 tablespoons soy sauce
- 1 tablespoon maple syrup
- 1 tablespoon lime juice
- 1 teaspoon grated ginger
- 1 clove of garlic, minced
- Water (as needed for desired consistency)

Instructions for Spring Rolls:

1. Fill a large shallow dish with warm water.
2. Dip one rice paper wrapper into the water for about 5 seconds until it softens.
3. Place the softened rice paper on a clean, damp kitchen towel.
4. In the center of the rice paper, layer a small amount of cooked rice vermicelli noodles, shredded lettuce, julienned carrots, cucumber, mint leaves, cilantro leaves, red bell pepper, and mango (if using).
5. Fold the sides of the rice paper over the filling and then roll it up tightly, similar to a burrito.
6. Repeat the process for the remaining rice paper wrappers and ingredients.

Instructions for Peanut Sauce:

1. In a small bowl, whisk together the creamy peanut butter, soy sauce, maple syrup, lime juice, grated ginger, and minced garlic.

2. Gradually add water to the peanut sauce, whisking until it reaches your desired dipping consistency.

3. Serve the rice paper spring rolls with the peanut sauce for dipping.

Vegan Stuffed Mushrooms

Ingredients:

- 20 large button mushrooms, stems removed and reserved
- 1 cup breadcrumbs (use gluten-free if needed)
- 1/2 cup finely chopped onion
- 2 cloves of garlic, minced
- 1/2 cup chopped spinach
- 1/4 cup chopped sun-dried tomatoes (rehydrated if dry)
- 1/4 cup chopped black olives
- 2 tablespoons nutritional yeast
- 2 tablespoons chopped fresh parsley

- 1 tablespoon olive oil

- Salt and pepper to taste

Instructions:

1. Preheat the oven to 375°F (190°C) and line a baking sheet with parchment paper.

2. Finely chop the reserved mushroom stems and set aside.

3. In a skillet, heat the olive oil over medium heat. Add the chopped onion and minced garlic, sauté until softened and fragrant.

4. Add the chopped mushroom stems, chopped spinach, sun-dried tomatoes, and chopped black olives to the skillet. Cook for another 2-3 minutes until the vegetables are tender.

5. Remove the skillet from the heat and stir in the breadcrumbs, nutritional yeast, chopped parsley, salt, and pepper.

6. Stuff each mushroom cap with the vegetable and breadcrumb mixture.

7. Place the stuffed mushrooms on the prepared baking sheet and bake in the preheated oven for 20-

25 minutes, or until the mushrooms are tender and the stuffing is golden brown.

Baked Sweet Potato Fries

Ingredients:

- 2 large sweet potatoes, peeled and cut into matchsticks
- 2 tablespoons olive oil
- 1 teaspoon paprika
- 1/2 teaspoon garlic powder
- 1/2 teaspoon onion powder
- Salt and pepper to taste

Instructions:

1. Preheat the oven to 425°F (220°C) and line a baking sheet with parchment paper.
2. In a large mixing bowl, toss the sweet potato matchsticks with olive oil, paprika, garlic powder, onion powder, salt, and pepper until well coated.
3. Spread the sweet potato fries in a single layer on the prepared baking sheet.

4. Bake in the preheated oven for 20-25 minutes, flipping the fries halfway through the cooking time, until they are crispy and golden brown.

5. Remove the baked sweet potato fries from the oven and serve immediately.

Vegan Buffalo Cauliflower Bites

Ingredients:

- 1 medium cauliflower, cut into bite-sized florets
- 1/2 cup all-purpose flour (use gluten-free flour if needed)
- 1/2 cup plant-based milk (almond, soy, or oat milk)
- 1 teaspoon garlic powder
- 1 teaspoon onion powder
- 1 teaspoon paprika
- 1/2 teaspoon salt
- 1/4 teaspoon black pepper
- 1/2 cup hot sauce (choose a vegan variety)
- 2 tablespoons melted vegan butter
- Ranch or blue cheese dressing (vegan) for dipping

Instructions:

1. Preheat the oven to 450°F (230°C) and line a baking
   sheet with parchment paper.

2. In a large mixing bowl, whisk together the all-
   purpose flour, plant-based milk, garlic powder,
   onion powder, paprika, salt, and black pepper until
   a smooth batter forms.

3. Dip each cauliflower floret into the batter, ensuring
   it's fully coated, and then shake off the excess.

4. Place the coated cauliflower florets on the prepared
   baking sheet in a single layer.

5. Bake in the preheated oven for 20-25 minutes, or
   until the cauliflower is tender and the batter is
   crispy.

6. In a separate bowl, combine the hot sauce and
   melted vegan butter. Toss the baked cauliflower
   bites in the sauce until evenly coated.

7. Return the coated cauliflower bites to the baking
   sheet and bake for an additional 5 minutes to set the
   sauce.

8. Serve the vegan buffalo cauliflower bites with ranch
   or blue cheese dressing for dipping.

Cucumber Avocado Sushi Rolls

Ingredients:

- 2 cups sushi rice

- 4 nori sheets

- 1 large cucumber, peeled and julienned

- 1 ripe avocado, sliced

- Pickled ginger, for serving (optional)

- Soy sauce or tamari, for dipping

Instructions:

1. Rinse the sushi rice in cold water until the water runs clear. Cook the rice according to the package instructions or using a rice cooker.

2. Lay a bamboo sushi rolling mat on a clean surface and place a nori sheet shiny side down on the mat.

3. Moisten your hands with water to prevent sticking, and then spread about 1/2 cup of cooked sushi rice evenly over the nori sheet, leaving a 1-inch border at the top.

4. Arrange cucumber juliennes and avocado slices in a line across the center of the rice.

5. Lift the edge of the bamboo mat closest to you and start rolling the sushi away from you, using gentle pressure to create a tight roll.

6. Wet the top border of the nori sheet with water to seal the roll.

7. Repeat the process for the remaining nori sheets and ingredients.

8. Once all the rolls are made, use a sharp knife to slice each roll into bite-sized pieces.

9. Serve the cucumber avocado sushi rolls with pickled ginger and soy sauce or tamari for dipping.

Vegan Bruschetta with Tomato and Basil

Ingredients:

- 1 French baguette, sliced
- 3 ripe tomatoes, diced
- 2 cloves of garlic, minced
- 1/4 cup fresh basil leaves, chopped
- 2 tablespoons balsamic vinegar
- 2 tablespoons extra-virgin olive oil

- Salt and pepper to taste

Instructions:
1. Preheat the oven to 375°F (190°C).
2. Arrange the sliced baguette on a baking sheet and lightly brush each slice with olive oil.
3. Toast the baguette slices in the preheated oven for 5-7 minutes or until they become crispy and lightly golden.
4. In a mixing bowl, combine the diced tomatoes, minced garlic, chopped basil leaves, balsamic vinegar, and extra-virgin olive oil.
5. Season the bruschetta mixture with salt and pepper to taste.
6. Spoon the tomato and basil mixture onto the toasted baguette slices.
7. Serve the vegan bruschetta as a delightful and refreshing appetizer.

Chapter 6: Desserts

In this chapter, we have presented a delightful assortment of ten vegan dessert recipes to satisfy your sweet cravings without compromising on health or dietary preferences.

Vegan Chocolate Avocado Mousse

Ingredients:

- 2 ripe avocados
- 1/2 cup unsweetened cocoa powder
- 1/3 cup maple syrup
- 1/4 cup almond milk
- 1 tsp vanilla extract
- A pinch of salt
- Fresh berries and mint leaves for garnish

Instructions:

1. In a food processor or blender, combine the ripe avocados, unsweetened cocoa powder, maple syrup, almond milk, vanilla extract, and a pinch of salt.

2. Blend until the mixture becomes smooth and creamy, scraping down the sides as needed.

3. Taste and adjust the sweetness if necessary by adding more maple syrup.

4. Transfer the mousse to serving glasses or bowls and refrigerate for at least 1 hour to set.

5. Before serving, garnish with fresh berries and mint leaves for an extra touch of freshness and color.

Vegan Banana Oat Cookies

Ingredients:

- 2 ripe bananas, mashed
- 1 1/2 cups rolled oats
- 1/4 cup almond butter
- 1/4 cup maple syrup
- 1 tsp vanilla extract
- 1/2 tsp ground cinnamon
- A pinch of salt
- 1/3 cup vegan chocolate chips (optional)

Instructions:

1. Preheat your oven to 350°F (175°C) and line a baking sheet with parchment paper.
2. In a large mixing bowl, combine the mashed bananas, rolled oats, almond butter, maple syrup, vanilla extract, ground cinnamon, and a pinch of salt.
3. Mix until all the ingredients are well combined.
4. If you want some extra indulgence, fold in the vegan chocolate chips into the cookie dough.
5. Scoop spoonfuls of the dough onto the prepared baking sheet and flatten them slightly with the back of a spoon.
6. Bake the cookies for about 12-15 minutes or until they turn golden brown around the edges.
7. Allow the cookies to cool on the baking sheet for a few minutes before transferring them to a wire rack to cool completely.

Vegan Blueberry Lemon Bars

Ingredients:

- 1 1/2 cups all-purpose flour
- 1/2 cup almond flour

- 1/2 cup coconut oil, softened
- 1/4 cup maple syrup
- Zest and juice of 1 lemon
- 1 tsp vanilla extract
- 1/2 tsp baking powder
- A pinch of salt
- 1 cup fresh blueberries

Instructions:

1. Preheat your oven to 350°F (175°C) and line an 8x8-inch baking pan with parchment paper.
2. In a mixing bowl, combine the all-purpose flour, almond flour, softened coconut oil, maple syrup, lemon zest, lemon juice, vanilla extract, baking powder, and a pinch of salt.
3. Mix until a crumbly dough forms.
4. Reserve about 1/2 cup of the dough and press the remaining dough evenly into the prepared baking pan to form the crust.
5. Spread the fresh blueberries evenly over the crust.
6. Crumble the reserved dough over the blueberries as the top layer.

7. Bake the bars for approximately 25-30 minutes or until the top turns golden brown.

8. Allow the bars to cool completely in the pan before cutting them into squares.

Chia Seed Chocolate Pudding

Ingredients:

- 1/4 cup chia seeds
- 1 1/2 cups almond milk
- 2 tbsp unsweetened cocoa powder
- 2 tbsp maple syrup
- 1 tsp vanilla extract
- A pinch of salt
- Fresh berries and chopped nuts for topping

Instructions:

1. In a jar or bowl, combine the chia seeds, almond milk, unsweetened cocoa powder, maple syrup, vanilla extract, and a pinch of salt.

2. Stir well until all the ingredients are thoroughly mixed.

3. Refrigerate the mixture for at least 3-4 hours or preferably overnight, allowing the chia seeds to absorb the liquid and create a pudding-like texture.

4. Before serving, give the pudding a good stir and top with fresh berries and chopped nuts for added flavor and texture.

Vegan Apple Crisp

Ingredients:

- 4 large apples, peeled, cored, and sliced
- 1 cup rolled oats
- 1/2 cup almond flour
- 1/4 cup maple syrup
- 1/4 cup coconut oil, melted
- 1 tsp ground cinnamon
- A pinch of salt
- Vegan vanilla ice cream or coconut whipped cream for serving (optional)

Instructions:

1. Preheat your oven to 350°F (175°C) and grease a 9x9-inch baking dish with coconut oil.

2. In a large mixing bowl, combine the sliced apples, rolled oats, almond flour, maple syrup, melted coconut oil, ground cinnamon, and a pinch of salt.

3. Toss the ingredients until the apples are evenly coated with the oat mixture.

4. Transfer the apple mixture to the prepared baking dish and spread it out evenly.

5. Bake the apple crisp for about 35-40 minutes or until the topping turns golden brown and the apples are tender.

6. Serve the apple crisp warm, and if desired, top it with vegan vanilla ice cream or coconut whipped cream for a delightful treat.

Almond Butter Energy Bites

Ingredients:

- 1 cup rolled oats
- 1/2 cup almond butter
- 1/3 cup maple syrup
- 1/4 cup vegan chocolate chips
- 1/4 cup shredded coconut
- 1 tsp vanilla extract

- A pinch of salt

Instructions:

1. In a mixing bowl, combine the rolled oats, almond butter, maple syrup, vegan chocolate chips, shredded coconut, vanilla extract, and a pinch of salt.
2. Mix well until all the ingredients are evenly distributed.
3. Take small portions of the mixture and roll them into bite-sized balls using your hands.
4. Place the energy bites on a parchment-lined tray and refrigerate for at least 30 minutes to firm up.
5. Once they are set, transfer the almond butter energy bites to an airtight container and keep them refrigerated until ready to serve.

Vegan Raspberry Coconut Popsicles

Ingredients:

- 1 cup fresh or frozen raspberries
- 1 1/2 cups coconut milk
- 2 tbsp maple syrup

- 1 tsp vanilla extract
- 1/4 cup shredded coconut

Instructions:

1. In a blender, combine the raspberries, coconut milk, maple syrup, and vanilla extract.
2. Blend until you get a smooth and creamy mixture.
3. Stir in the shredded coconut into the raspberry coconut milk mixture.
4. Pour the mixture into popsicle molds and insert popsicle sticks.
5. Freeze the popsicles for at least 4-6 hours or until they are completely solid.
6. To remove the popsicles from the molds, run them under warm water for a few seconds, and they should slide out easily.

Vegan Carrot Cake Cupcakes

Ingredients:

- 1 1/2 cups grated carrots
- 1 cup all-purpose flour
- 1/2 cup almond flour

- 1/2 cup coconut sugar

- 1/4 cup maple syrup

- 1/4 cup coconut oil, melted

- 1/4 cup unsweetened applesauce

- 1 tsp baking powder

- 1/2 tsp baking soda

- 1 tsp ground cinnamon

- 1/2 tsp ground ginger

- A pinch of nutmeg

- A pinch of salt

- Vegan cream cheese frosting (store-bought or homemade) for topping

Instructions:

1. Preheat your oven to 350°F (175°C) and line a muffin tin with cupcake liners.

2. In a mixing bowl, combine the grated carrots, all-purpose flour, almond flour, coconut sugar, maple syrup, melted coconut oil, unsweetened applesauce, baking powder, baking soda, ground cinnamon, ground ginger, nutmeg, and a pinch of salt.

3. Stir until all the ingredients are well incorporated.

4. Spoon the batter into the cupcake liners, filling them about 2/3 full.

5. Bake the cupcakes for approximately 18-20 minutes or until a toothpick inserted in the center comes out clean.

6. Allow the cupcakes to cool completely before frosting them with vegan cream cheese frosting.

Dairy-Free Chocolate Fudge

Ingredients:

- 1 cup vegan chocolate chips
- 1/2 cup almond butter
- 1/4 cup coconut oil, melted
- 2 tbsp maple syrup
- 1 tsp vanilla extract
- A pinch of salt
- Chopped nuts or sea salt flakes for garnish (optional)

Instructions:

1. In a microwave-safe bowl or on the stove, melt the vegan chocolate chips until smooth.

2. Stir in the almond butter, melted coconut oil, maple syrup, vanilla extract, and a pinch of salt.

3. Mix until all the ingredients are well combined and you have a silky chocolate mixture.

4. Pour the fudge mixture into a parchment-lined 8x8-inch baking dish.

5. Smooth the top with a spatula and, if desired, sprinkle chopped nuts or sea salt flakes on top for extra flavor and texture.

6. Refrigerate the fudge for at least 1-2 hours to set.

7. Once the fudge is firm, cut it into squares and indulge in this delectable dairy-free treat.

Vegan Mango Sorbet

Ingredients:

- 3 ripe mangoes, peeled and diced
- 1/4 cup coconut milk
- 2 tbsp maple syrup
- 1 tsp lemon juice
- A pinch of salt

Instructions:

1. In a blender or food processor, combine the diced mangoes, coconut milk, maple syrup, lemon juice, and a pinch of salt.

2. Blend until you get a smooth and creamy sorbet mixture.

3. Transfer the sorbet mixture to a shallow dish or ice cream maker if you have one.

4. If using a shallow dish, cover it with a lid or cling wrap and freeze for at least 4 hours, stirring the sorbet every hour to prevent ice crystals from forming.

5. If using an ice cream maker, follow the manufacturer's instructions to churn the sorbet until it reaches the desired consistency.

6. Serve the vegan mango sorbet in chilled bowls or cones for a refreshing and naturally sweet dessert option.

Chapter 7: Smoothies

In this Chapter, we explore a delightful array of smoothie recipes that are not only vegan but also packed with essential nutrients, vitamins, and antioxidants. These smoothies are designed to cater to your taste buds while promoting your overall health and well-being. Whether you're looking for a refreshing green boost or a tropical twist, we've got you covered. So, let's dive into these nutritious concoctions and start blending our way to a healthier lifestyle!

Green Smoothie with Spinach and Kale:

Ingredients:

- 1 cup fresh spinach leaves
- 1 cup chopped kale
- 1 ripe banana
- 1/2 cucumber, peeled and diced
- 1 green apple, cored and sliced
- 1/2 cup coconut water

- 1 tablespoon chia seeds

- Ice cubes (optional)

Instructions:

1. Place the spinach, kale, banana, cucumber, and green apple in a blender.
2. Add the coconut water and chia seeds.
3. Blend on high until smooth and creamy.
4. If desired, add a few ice cubes and blend again.
5. Pour into a glass and enjoy the refreshing goodness of this green smoothie!

Vegan Berry Blast Smoothie:

Ingredients:

- 1 cup mixed berries (strawberries, blueberries, raspberries)

- 1 ripe banana

- 1/2 cup almond milk

- 1 tablespoon hemp seeds

- 1 tablespoon maple syrup (optional)

- Fresh mint leaves for garnish

Instructions:

1. Combine the mixed berries, banana, almond milk, and hemp seeds in a blender.
2. If you prefer a sweeter taste, add a drizzle of maple syrup.
3. Blend until the mixture reaches a smooth consistency.
4. Pour into a glass and garnish with fresh mint leaves.
5. Sip on this delightful berry blast and let the flavors dance on your palate!

Tropical Turmeric Smoothie:

Ingredients:

- 1 cup fresh pineapple chunks
- 1 ripe mango, peeled and diced
- 1 small orange, peeled and segmented
- 1/2-inch piece of fresh ginger, peeled
- 1/2 teaspoon ground turmeric
- 1 cup coconut water
- 1 tablespoon flaxseeds

Instructions:

1. Place the pineapple chunks, mango, orange segments, and ginger in the blender.

2. Add the ground turmeric and coconut water.

3. Blend until the mixture is smooth and creamy.

4. Sprinkle flaxseeds on top and give it a gentle stir.

5. Savor the taste of the tropics with this invigorating turmeric smoothie!

Vegan Chocolate Banana Smoothie:

Ingredients:

- 2 ripe bananas
- 2 tablespoons unsweetened cocoa powder
- 1 cup almond milk
- 1 tablespoon almond butter
- 1 teaspoon vanilla extract
- 1 tablespoon maple syrup (optional)
- Dark chocolate shavings for garnish

Instructions:

1. Peel and slice the ripe bananas.

2. In the blender, combine the banana slices, cocoa powder, almond milk, almond butter, and vanilla extract.

3. For added sweetness, drizzle in a bit of maple syrup if desired.

4. Blend until the mixture becomes thick and creamy.

5. Pour the smoothie into a glass, garnish with dark chocolate shavings, and relish the chocolaty goodness!

Vegan Peanut Butter and Banana Smoothie:

Ingredients:

- 2 ripe bananas
- 2 tablespoons peanut butter (unsweetened and no added oil)
- 1 cup oat milk
- 1 tablespoon flaxseeds
- 1 tablespoon agave nectar (optional)
- Crushed peanuts for topping

Instructions:

1. Peel and slice the ripe bananas.

2. In the blender, combine the banana slices, peanut butter, oat milk, and flaxseeds.

3. If you prefer a sweeter taste, add a drizzle of agave nectar.

4. Blend until the mixture reaches a creamy consistency.

5. Pour into a glass, top with crushed peanuts, and indulge in the nutty deliciousness!

Beetroot and Berry Smoothie:

Ingredients:

- 1 small beetroot, peeled and diced
- 1 cup mixed berries (strawberries, raspberries, blackberries)
- 1/2 cup coconut water
- 1 tablespoon chia seeds
- 1 tablespoon agave nectar (optional)
- Fresh mint leaves for garnish

Instructions:

1. Place the diced beetroot and mixed berries in the blender.

2. Add the coconut water and chia seeds.

3. For a touch of sweetness, drizzle in a bit of agave nectar if desired.

4. Blend until the mixture turns into a vibrant, smooth concoction.

5. Pour the smoothie into a glass, garnish with fresh mint leaves, and savor the earthy-sweet fusion of flavors!

Vegan Mango Lassi Smoothie:

Ingredients:

- 2 ripe mangoes, peeled and diced
- 1 cup coconut yogurt
- 1/2 cup almond milk
- 1/2 teaspoon ground cardamom
- 1 tablespoon maple syrup (optional)
- Chopped pistachios for topping

Instructions:

1. In the blender, combine the diced mangoes, coconut yogurt, almond milk, and ground cardamom.

2. If you prefer a touch of sweetness, add a drizzle of maple syrup.

3. Blend until the mixture becomes creamy and luscious.

4. Pour the smoothie into a glass, top with chopped pistachios, and delight in this Indian-inspired mango lassi!

Blueberry Almond Smoothie:

Ingredients:

- 1 cup fresh blueberries
- 1 ripe banana
- 1 cup almond milk
- 1 tablespoon almond butter
- 1 tablespoon honey or agave nectar (optional)
- Sliced almonds for topping

Instructions:

1. Combine the fresh blueberries, ripe banana, almond milk, and almond butter in the blender.

2. For added sweetness, drizzle in a bit of honey or agave nectar if desired.

3. Blend until the mixture turns velvety and rich.

4. Pour into a glass, top with sliced almonds, and indulge in the nutty-berry goodness!

Vegan Kale and Pineapple Smoothie:

Ingredients:

- 1 cup chopped kale
- 1 cup fresh pineapple chunks
- 1 ripe banana
- 1/2 cup coconut water
- 1 tablespoon hemp seeds
- 1 tablespoon lime juice
- Ice cubes (optional)

Instructions:

1. Place the chopped kale, pineapple chunks, ripe banana, and coconut water in the blender.

2. Add the hemp seeds and lime juice.

3. If you prefer a chilled smoothie, toss in a few ice cubes before blending.

4. Blend until the mixture becomes a luscious, green elixir.

5. Pour into a glass and enjoy the tropical-kale fusion!

Creamy Avocado and Spinach Smoothie:

Ingredients:

- 1 ripe avocado, peeled and pitted
- 1 cup fresh spinach leaves
- 1 cup almond milk
- 1 tablespoon agave nectar or maple syrup
- 1 tablespoon lime juice
- Pinch of salt
- Fresh basil leaves for garnish

Instructions:

1. In the blender, combine the ripe avocado, fresh spinach leaves, almond milk, agave nectar (or maple syrup), lime juice, and a pinch of salt.

2. Blend until the mixture becomes creamy and luscious.

3. Pour the smoothie into a glass and garnish with fresh basil leaves.

4. Sip on this creamy avocado and spinach smoothie and relish its velvety texture!

CONCLUSION

As we reach the final chapter of this guide, it is essential to reflect on the journey we have taken together in exploring the realm of easy vegan recipes tailored specifically for individuals managing diabetes and kidney disease. Throughout these pages, we have delved into the profound impact a plant-based diet can have on one's overall health and well-being, particularly when faced with these challenging conditions.

I would like to emphasize that the information presented here is not just an amalgamation of generic advice, but rather a thoughtful compilation of evidence-based research, expert insights, and personal experiences from those who have successfully embraced the vegan lifestyle while battling diabetes and kidney issues. My intention has been to provide you with an authentic resource that serves as a compass guiding you towards better health.

Throughout the preceding chapters, we have seen the potential benefits of adopting a vegan diet. From nutrient-rich breakfast options like Vegan Blueberry Chia Seed Pudding and Tofu Scramble with Spinach and Tomatoes to satisfying lunch choices such as Lentil and Vegetable Soup and Vegan Chickpea Salad Sandwich, and ending with delectable dinners like Vegan Lentil Shepherd's Pie and Cauliflower and Chickpea Curry, each recipe has been meticulously selected to cater to your health needs without compromising on taste.

Moreover, I want to underscore that this guide is not meant to replace professional medical advice. While a vegan diet can be beneficial for many individuals managing diabetes and kidney disease, it is crucial to consult with a qualified healthcare provider before making any significant dietary changes. Your doctor will help personalize the recommendations based on your unique medical history, current health status, and individual nutritional requirements.

As we conclude this journey together, I encourage you to view this guide as a stepping stone rather than an endpoint. Embrace this newfound knowledge and use it to explore the vast array of plant-based culinary delights that await you. The world of vegan cuisine is dynamic and ever-evolving, with innovative recipes and creative chefs continuously pushing the boundaries of what is possible.

Beyond the recipes shared here, I encourage you to experiment with ingredients, spices, and flavors, allowing your creativity to flourish in the kitchen. Engaging in this culinary adventure can not only make the process of preparing meals enjoyable but can also lead to delightful surprises and discoveries that enrich your dining experience.

In closing, I want to express my gratitude for allowing me to be a part of your quest for a healthier life. My hope is that this guide has provided you with practical tools, inspiration, and a sense of empowerment to make informed choices that positively impact your health and well-being. Remember that each small step taken towards a plant-based diet is a step towards better health, not just for yourself but also for the environment.

As you embrace the power of plant-based nutrition, I wish you success in your journey towards managing diabetes and kidney disease with compassion, resilience, and joy. May your kitchen become a sanctuary of health and happiness, and may your heart be filled with gratitude for the abundance that nature offers.

Thank you for embarking on this adventure with me, and remember, the path to wellness is a continuous one. Keep learning, exploring, and nourishing both your body and soul. Be kind to yourself and others, and may your life be filled with vibrant health and prosperity.

Farewell and bon appétit!